SILDENAFIL FOR BEGINNERS GUIDE

THE DOCTORS GUIDE FOR ELIMINATING ERECTILE DYSFUNCTION OR IMPOTENCE TO ENABLE MEN LAST LONGER AND HARDER TO MAKE HER SCREAM

ANJANA SHETH

Copyright © Anjana Sheth
All Rights Reserved.

This book has been self-published with all reasonable efforts taken to make the material error-free by the author. No part of this book shall be used, reproduced in any manner whatsoever without written permission from the author, except in the case of brief quotations embodied in critical articles and reviews.

The Author of this book is solely responsible and liable for its content including but not limited to the views, representations, descriptions, statements, information, opinions and references ["Content"]. The Content of this book shall not constitute or be construed or deemed to reflect the opinion or expression of the Publisher or Editor. Neither the Publisher nor Editor endorse or approve the Content of this book or guarantee the reliability, accuracy or completeness of the Content published herein and do not make any representations or warranties of any kind, express or implied, including but not limited to the implied warranties of merchantability, fitness for a particular purpose. The Publisher and Editor shall not be liable whatsoever for any errors, omissions, whether such errors or omissions result from negligence, accident, or any other cause or claims for loss or damages of any kind, including without limitation, indirect or consequential loss or damage arising out of use, inability to use, or about the reliability, accuracy or sufficiency of the information contained in this book.

Made with ♥ on the Notion Press Platform
www.notionpress.com

Contents

Title Page	v
1. Introduction	1
2. Earlier Than Sildenafil	2
3. Tips On Using Sildenafil	3
4. Is There Any Risk	5
5. Sildenafil Explained	7
6. About Sildenafil	15
The End	21

Title Page

SILDENAFIL FOR BEGINNERS GUIDE

The Doctors Guide for Eliminating Erectile Dysfunction or Impotence to Enable Men Last Longer and Harder to Make Her Scream

Anjana Sheth

Copyright@2022

CHAPTER ONE

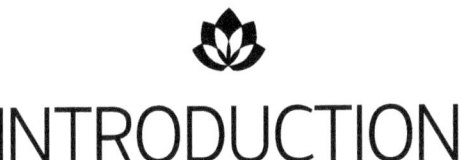

INTRODUCTION

Having erectile dysfunction, often known as impotence, implies that you have trouble getting or keeping an erection. The most frequent reason is a constriction of the arteries supplying blood to the penis, although there are other reasons as well.

Sildenafil blocks the enzyme phosphodiesterase type 5 in the body, hence improving erectile dysfunction. This aids in the dilation (relaxation) of blood vessels, which increases blood flow to the penis after an intercourse. This aids in keeping an erection going strong.

One may get sildenafil with a doctor's prescription. Branded Viagra® is exclusively accessible on the NHS for men with erectile dysfunction caused by specific medical conditions, but non-branded (generic) pills of sildenafil are available to everyone.

Sildenafil is also available without a prescription from certain pharmacies. Find out if this choice is right for you from your pharmacy.

To learn more about the use of Revatio®, a different brand of sildenafil tablets, in the treatment of pulmonary arterial hypertension, please refer to the patient information sheet titled Sildenafil for pulmonary hypertension.

CHAPTER TWO

Earlier than sildenafil

In some cases, a patient may be able to take a medication, but only if special precautions are taken. These are some things you should tell your doctor before starting sildenafil:

If your penis is injured, sick, or otherwise messed up in any way, treatment may be necessary.

If you suffer from cardiovascular disease or vascular illness.

If you're legally blind because of an eye problem.

In the event that you suffer from angina or low blood pressure.

If you're experiencing any issues with your kidneys or liver.

If you have a bleeding disorder, such a stomach ulcer.

If sickle cell illness affects you.

If you have a history of leukemia or cancer of the bone marrow.

If you're utilizing any other medications. All over-the-counter medications, supplements, and illegal substances are included here.

If you have ever had a medication-related adverse reaction.

CHAPTER THREE

Tips on using sildenafil

The manufacturer recommends reading the included pamphlet with information on sildenafil before to use. It will supply you with further details on the pills and a comprehensive list of potential adverse reactions.

Follow your healthcare provider's instructions while taking sildenafil. It should be taken before to engaging in sexual activity; it is NOT meant for everyday usage. One tablet should be taken approximately an hour before sexual activity is anticipated, while its effectiveness may be maintained for up to five hours following ingestion. The pill may be taken before or after eating, however its effectiveness may be diminished if taken soon after a very substantial meal.

Tablets of sildenafil come in three different dosages: 25 mg, 50 mg, and 100 mg. You'll probably start out with a 50-milligram pill and have your dosage adjusted from there based on how your body responds. Be sure that the pill strength you were anticipating is in the bottle each time you pick up a prescription.

Never take more than one dosage of sildenafil in a 24-hour period.

Maximizing the Benefits of Medical Care

Foreplay is still necessary whether or not you are taking medication for erectile dysfunction. Sildenafil won't work to get you horny unless you're already in the mood to get one.

Don't pound the booze before popping a sildenafil pill. You may not receive the full advantage of the pills if you drink alcohol, which might impair your ability to achieve an erection.

Don't mix sildenafil with grapefruit juice, since it might have adverse effects. This is because grapefruit juice contains a substance that might increase the quantity of sildenafil in your system, increasing the likelihood of adverse effects.

Be sure to keep all of your checkups with the doctor so that your recovery can be closely monitored. You should tell your doctor if you find the strength of the pills to be too much for you. Do not take more pills than your doctor has prescribed if you do not develop an erection after taking sildenafil or if it does not last long enough for you to have sex.

Sildenafil should not be used in conjunction with any other treatment for erectile dysfunction.

CHAPTER FOUR

Is there any risk

The majority of medications include undesirable side effects along with their beneficial ones, however not everyone feels them. Some of the most frequent side effects of sildenafil are included in the table below. See the manufacturer's information booklet that came with your medication for a complete list. There is usually a decrease in negative effects as your body adapts to the new medication, but if any of the following persist or become bothersome, you should contact your doctor or pharmacist.

Regular users of sildenafil might expect to experience a number of well-known negative effects (these affect more than 1 in 10 men)

Headache

Take in plenty of fluids. In the event that your headaches persist, you should see a medical professional.

Consequences of sildenafil that are all too common (these affect fewer than 1 in 10 men)

In this event, what should I do?

Dizziness, nausea, bloatedness, and a clogged nose

symptoms include dizziness, altered vision (including blurring or distorted colors), and nausea

Do not operate heavy machinery or drive a vehicle until your eyesight and reflexes have returned to normal after experiencing any of these conditions.

Warning: seek immediate medical assistance if your erection lasts more than four hours, you have chest discomfort, or you suddenly lose your eyesight.

See your physician or pharmacist if you have any additional concerns about side effects from the pills.

Storing Sildenafil Properly

Every medication should be stored where children cannot have access to them.

Keep out of the reach of both heat and light by storing in a cold, dry area.

CHAPTER FIVE

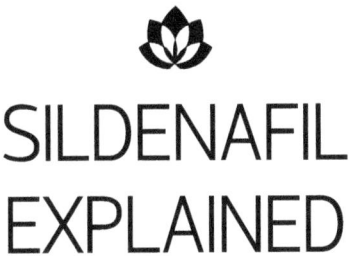

SILDENAFIL EXPLAINED

Where does this medication fit in?

The condition of erectile dysfunction may be remedied with its help (ED).

Treatment of pulmonary hypertension using this drug.

You could get it for some other purpose. Consult your physician.

When should I notify my doctor that I am allergic to this drug?

For any and all applications of the drug:

In the event that you have previously been diagnosed with an allergy to this medication, any of its components, or any other medications, foods, or substances. Explain to your doctor what symptoms you experienced.

Diseases like pulmonary veno-occlusive disease are very serious and may cause death (PVOD).

Use of "popper" substances like amyl nitrite and butyl nitrite.

Any of the following should be avoided if you are currently taking any of the following medications: Nitroglycerin, riociguat, ritonavir, vericiguat, and isosorbide dinitrate or mononitrate.

If you're on the antifungal medications itraconazole or ketoconazole, then you should avoid eating mushrooms.

If you are already taking a medication that has the same active ingredient.

If you are currently using another medication for ED or hypertension, you should not use this one.

If you're experiencing problems with getting an erection, try these:

In the event that you have been informed that your health prevents you from engaging in sexual activity.

For the ladies among us. For that reason, female patients are not permitted to use this medication.

In the case of a pediatric patient. It has been determined that this medication is neither safe or suitable for usage in children.

No attempt has been made to include all possible drug–health interactions for this medication.

Share all of your medication history with your doctor and pharmacist, including over-the-counter medications, herbal supplements, and prescription pharmaceuticals. You should determine whether or not the use of this medication may interact negatively with any other medications you are currently taking or health conditions you have. Do not alter your treatment plan, including the timing of any dosage adjustments or the introduction of new medications, without first consulting your physician.

When I'm under the influence of this medication, what should I keep in mind?

For any and all applications of the drug:

You should let all of your doctors know that you are taking this medication. This covers all of your visits to the clinic, hospital, pharmacy, and dentist.

Until you know how this medication affects you, stay away from the wheel and any other activities that need your full attention.

If you have been sitting or laying down, get up gently to prevent dizziness and fainting. If you must use the stairs, please do so with caution.

Before starting an alcohol regimen, discuss it with your doctor.

Occasionally, this medication has been linked to adverse events such as irregular heartbeat, heart attack, stroke, pulmonary hemorrhage, and very high blood pressure. This has resulted in death on occasion. These adverse effects occurred more often in patients who already had heart disease before starting this medication. The drug's role in triggering these side effects is unknown. Get in touch with your physician if you have any concerns or inquiries.

Very serious eye problems have occurred extremely seldom with this medicine. Changes to or complete loss of one's vision may result from this, and in some cases the damage may be permanent. Consult your physician.

Consult your physician if you have sickle cell disease.

Take caution while using this medication if you are 65 or older. There may be further complications.

If you're experiencing problems with getting an erection, try these:

The transmission of sexually transmitted illnesses such as HIV and hepatitis is not impeded by this medication. Use a latex or polyurethane condom every time you have intercourse.

Chronically elevated pulmonary arterial pressure:

It has been determined that this medication is neither safe or suitable for usage in children. The pediatric mortality rate increases with increasing doses of this medication. The doctor treating your child must assess the potential advantages of giving this medication to your kid against any potential drawbacks. Discuss the potential advantages and disadvantages of this medication with your child's doctor if he or she has been prescribed it. If you're concerned about providing this medicine to your kid, consult with a medical professional.

If you are pregnant, trying to become pregnant, or currently breastfeeding, you should let your doctor know. You and your unborn child need to weigh the pros and cons of this decision.

What are some immediate symptoms I should report to my doctor?

WARNING/CAUTION: Some persons using a medicine may have serious and even fatal adverse effects, however this is very uncommon. If you have any of the following symptoms, which may be associated with a severe adverse impact, you should contact your doctor or seek emergency medical attention immediately.

Allergic reactions manifest themselves with symptoms such as a rash, hives, itching, red, swollen, blistered, or peeling skin (with or without fever), wheezing, chest tightness, difficulty breathing, swallowing, or speaking, unusual hoarseness, and swelling of the mouth, face, lips, tongue, and throat.

Pressure or soreness in the chest.

Beats the heart too quickly or irregularly.

Feeling faint or dizzy.

Abnormally queasy or sick to one's stomach.

symptoms such as numbness or tingling in one or both hands, difficulty speaking or thinking, a shift in balance, a sagging of the face on one side, or a loss of peripheral vision on one eye.

Observational shift in visual perception.
Impairment of vision.
Hearing loss, tinnitus, and other auditory disturbances.
The breathing difficulty is new, perhaps much worse.
Arm or leg swelling.
Fever.
Strange cuts, bruises, or bleeding that can't be explained.

If you get a painful erection (hard penis) or an erection that lasts more than 4 hours, it is important to see your doctor immediately. This is possible even if you are not sexually active. You risk permanent inability to have sex if this is not addressed soon away.

We need to know whether there are any additional potential risks associated with this medication.

Every medication has the potential to induce unwanted side effects. However many individuals report no or minimal negative reactions to the drug. If any of the following adverse effects, or any others, cause you concern or do not go away, you should see a medical professional.

For any and all applications of the drug:
Flushing.
Headache.
Heartburn.
The stomach was upset.
congested or runny nose.
hurting muscles.

If you're experiencing problems with getting an erection, try these:
That hurts my back.
Chronically elevated pulmonary arterial pressure:
Diarrhea.
Redness.

Nosebleed.

Sleep disturbances.

The potential adverse effects listed here are not exhaustive. See your physician if any unwanted effects persist. If you're experiencing adverse affects, see your doctor right away.

Report any adverse affects to your country's health department.

Get in touch with the Food and Drug Administration at 1-800-332-1088 if you have any adverse reactions. In addition, adverse reactions may be reported at https://www.fda.gov/medwatch.

What is the recommended dosage for this medication?

Listen to your doctor's advice and take this medication as prescribed. Keep in mind what you've been told.

Regardless of whether you take it with or without meals, you should take any oral medication.

If you suffer from erectile dysfunction (ED), take this medication 30 minutes before engaging in sexual activity. Discuss your dosing schedule with your doctor if you have any questions.

Take just the amount prescribed by your doctor. Keep from using more often or for longer than prescribed. Increasing the likelihood of really harmful side effects is possible if you do any of these activities.

Maintain taking this medication as directed by your doctor or other healthcare practitioner for high pulmonary arterial pressure even if you feel OK.

Shake the suspension (liquid) thoroughly before using.

Be precise while dosing liquids. Please make use of the medication's included measurement tool.

It is administered by injecting it directly into a vein.

Just what should I do if I forget to take my medication?

To treat ED, this medication is used just as required. Don't take more than what the doctor prescribes.

Take just one dosage each day.

When dealing with pulmonary hypertension, a missing dosage should be taken as soon as it is remembered.

If it is almost time for your next dosage, do not take the one you missed.

Please don't double up on your dosages or take more than what was prescribed.

Injections: See your physician for instructions.

Please advise on the proper methods for stowing and disposing of this medication.

Keep at room temperature or in the fridge if it's a liquid (suspension). Be sure you don't freeze over.

Keep dry while storing. A bathroom is not a suitable storage location.

60 days after preparation, discard any unneeded portion of this medicine. If you are unsure of when this is, see your pharmacist.

A bathroom is not a suitable storage location.

You should discuss the best way to keep your injectable medication at home with your doctor, nurse, or pharmacist.

Any and all goods:

Don't leave any drugs lying about. All medications should be stored safely, out of the reach of children and animals.

Drugs that have expired or are no longer needed should be discarded. Do not put anything down a drain or flush a toilet unless instructed to. If you have concerns about how to properly dispose of medication, see your pharmacist. There might be local drug return programs available.

A Few Facts About Drugs in General

It's important to see a doctor if your symptoms persist or worsen.

Don't give other people drugs and don't accept drugs from other people.

Additional drug leaflets may be available for certain medications. Talk to your doctor, nurse, pharmacist, or other healthcare professional if you have any concerns or questions regarding this medication.

There may be a different drug-specific leaflet available for certain medications. Make sure you ask the pharmacist. Please consult your physician, nurse, pharmacist, or other healthcare professional with any questions or concerns you may have about the use of this medication.

Call your local poison control center or go to the hospital if you fear someone has overdosed. Go ready to describe the stolen items, their values, and the time frame in which they were taken.

CHAPTER SIX

ABOUT SILDENAFIL

Phosphodiesterase type-5 (PDE 5) inhibitors, of which SILDENAFIL is a member, are often prescribed to adult males for the treatment of erectile dysfunction (impotence). In addition, SILDENAFIL may be used to treat people with pulmonary arterial hypertension (high blood pressure in the lungs) to enhance exercise tolerance and reduce the progression of the disease.

When a person is sexually aroused, SILDENAFIL causes the blood vessels in the penis to relax, enabling more blood to flow into the penis. Erectile dysfunction may be treated with SILDENAFIL. The blood vessel-relaxing effect of SILDENAFIL improves oxygen delivery to the lungs and eases the strain on the heart. Effectively managing pulmonary hypertension as a result.

Depending on your medical condition, your doctor may recommend taking SILDENAFIL for an extended period of time. Headache, nausea, dizziness, indigestion, and stomach trouble are some of the negative effects that have been reported by those using SILDENAFIL. These unwanted effects often disappear without any medical intervention and quickly. Nonetheless, if you see any of these symptoms persisting, it's best to consult your doctor.

You should not use SILDENAFIL if you have an allergy to any of the ingredients or if you are also taking nitrate medications or riociguat (a drug used to treat pulmonary hypertension). Children should not take SILDENAFIL. If your hearing or eyesight is deteriorating, you should see a doctor. Stay away from alcoholic beverages since they might hinder your capacity to obtain an erection. It is recommended that SILDENAFIL be taken with light meals since it may take longer for the drug to act if taken after a large meal.

SILDENAFIL is used for pulmonary arterial hypertension and erectile dysfunction (impotence).

Health Advantages

To treat erectile dysfunction (impotence) in adult men and pulmonary arterial hypertension (high blood pressure in the lungs) in adults to enhance exercise tolerance and slow clinical worsening, SILDENAFIL is prescribed as a member of the class of drugs known as phosphodiesterase type-5 (PDE 5) inhibitors. When a person is sexually aroused, SILDENAFIL causes the blood vessels in the penis to relax, enabling more blood to flow into the penis. Nevertheless, SILDENAFIL aids in obtaining an erection only if the individual is sexually aroused. The blood vessel-relaxing effect of SILDENAFIL improves oxygen delivery to the lungs and eases the strain on the heart. Effectively treating pulmonary hypertension as a result.

Tips for Using

Tablet/Capsule: To take it, just chew it up and down a full glass of water. Do not alter the shape of the tablet by crushing, breaking, or chewing. If the product is a syrup or suspension, shake it up before using. Use the measuring cup included in the package to administer the recommended dosage. An Oral Suspension Powder: Before using, make sure you read the label. To prepare, fill the container with the recommended amount of water, replace the lid, and shake vigorously for 30 seconds. Make sure you use the dosage syringe to get the right amount of medicine. Sachet: Cut open the packet and eat everything inside. Keep the strip in your mouth until it dissolves, since this is how an orally disintegrating strip works. Avoid gulping it down whole. Keep your hands dry if you need to handle the strip. Jelly: Dissolve jelly by placing it in your mouth or beneath your tongue. Effervescent tablets: Follow the guidelines on the packaging or your doctor's advice. Effervescent tablets should be taken by dissolving one in half a glass of water and drinking the resulting solution right away.

Storage

To avoid damage, keep out of direct sunlight and in a cool, dry environment.

Sildenafil's headache-inducing side effects

Nausea

Dizziness

Indigestion

GI distress

Detailed Cautionary Statement and Warn

Cautionary Statements About Drugs

Do not use SILDENAFIL if you have ever had an adverse reaction to any of the ingredients, if you are currently taking any medications that stimulate the guanylate cyclase enzyme, or if you have ever had angina or chest discomfort while taking nitrates (used to treat heart failure and PAH). If you suffer from or have ever suffered from angina, a heart attack, an irregular heartbeat, heart failure, poor blood circulation, low blood pressure, eye or ear problems, sickle cell anemia (a red blood cell abnormality), multiple myeloma (bone marrow cancer), leukemia (blood cancer), a stomach ulcer, bleeding problems, problems with the shape of the genitalia, or Peyronie's disease, you should tell your doctor (a condition that causes painful erections).

Interactions Between Medications

Interactions with Other Drugs: SILDENAFIL may interact with nitrate medications (nitroglycerin), guanylate cyclase stimulators (riociguat), protease inhibitors (ritonavir), anti-fungal medications (ketoconazole, itraconazole), and alpha-blockers/anti-hypertensive medications.

Taking SILDENAFIL after a large meal might delay the medicine's effects, so it's best to take the medication with a small meal. If you want to maintain your capacity to acquire an erection, it's best to avoid alcohol.

Warning: Tell your doctor if you have or have had had heart disease, high blood pressure, stomach ulcers, bleeding disorders, a deformed penis, or Peyronie's disease since these conditions may interact with certain medications (a condition that causes painful erections).

Lifestyle and Eating Tips

Managing erectile dysfunction may be facilitated by maintaining a healthy weight, eating a balanced diet, and engaging in regular exercise.

Don't drink alcohol if you want to keep your erections healthy.

Don't smoke cigarettes.

Spend time together in a sexually intimate way.

Warning! Extraordinary Advice

If you have been given SILDENAFIL to treat erectile dysfunction, take it no more than once daily.

If the erection lasts more than four hours following sexual activity, you should see a doctor.

Disorders and Illnesses Worry Patients Glossary

Impotence or impotence: An inability to maintain a firm, erect penis necessary for sexual activity. Stress, worry, melancholy, poor self-esteem, and a fear of sexual failure are all possible causes. Erectile dysfunction is exacerbated by lifestyle and health variables such smoking, drinking, obesity, inactivity, and high blood pressure. Erectile dysfunction is characterized by issues with achieving and maintaining an erection, as well as a lack of motivation to engage in sexual activity.

The arteries in the lungs and heart are negatively impacted by high blood pressure, which leads to pulmonary arterial hypertension (PAH). Caused by constricted blood arteries, which provide extra strain on the heart. You may have discomfort in the chest, lightheadedness, weariness, and swelling in the feet and legs.

The End